Udder health

It is a proven fact that many cases of clinical mastitis that arise during the first 100 days of lactation are caused by IMIs that have occurred over the dry period, or IMIs that have persisted throughout the dry period. More than 50 % of cases of clinical mastitis caused by coliform bacteria in the first 100 days of lactation arise from an IMI developed during the dry period. Intramammary infections that develop at the beginning of the dry period and are caused by environmental streptococci are responsible for 36 % of clinical mastitis cases at calving. These IMIs persist until the next lactation in 55 % of cases.

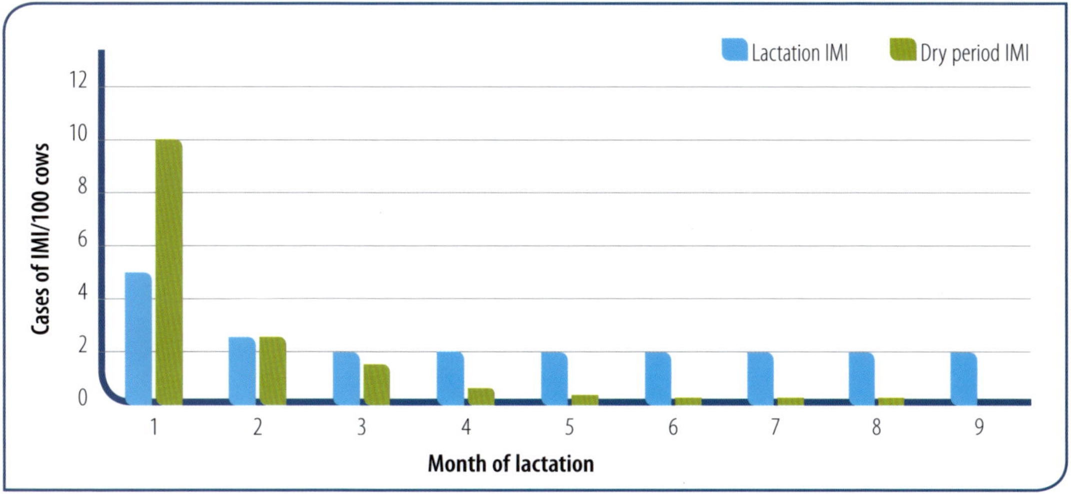

Figure 1. Origin of intramammary infections (lactation or dry period) in cases of clinical mastitis. Data adapted from Green et al., 2002.

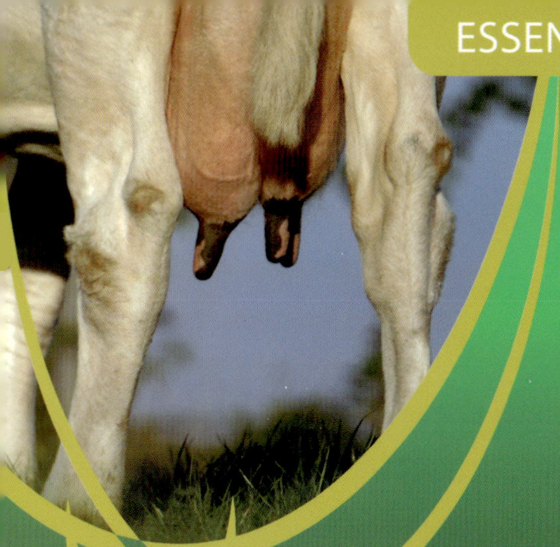

ESSENTIAL GUIDES ON CATTLE FARMING

Drying-Off Management

Luis Miguel Jiménez Galán

SERVET

"Dedicated to Juan Carlos Bravo, friend and colleague, and a great visionary in the dairy sector. We will miss you."

The author

Luís Miguel Jiménez Galán

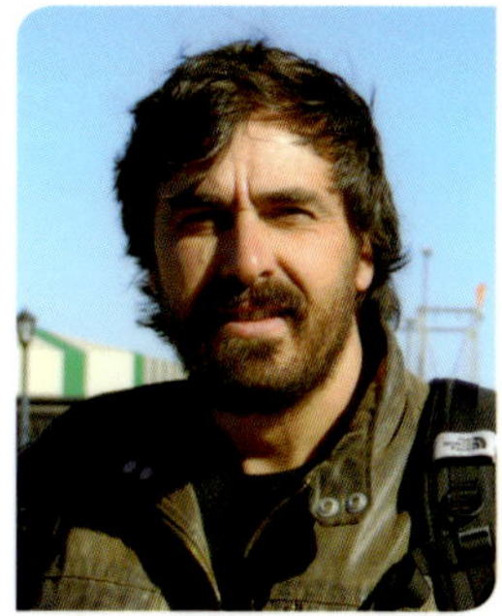

Degree in veterinary medicine from the Complutense University of Madrid (Spain) in 1992. Director of SERVET TALAVERA S.L., an international company specialised in milk quality and mastitis control. Speaker in various arenas (National Mastitis Council, International Dairy Federation, Spanish Association of Bovine Medicine Specialists) and dairy consultant in over 15 countries. He has been vice president and spokesman for milk quality at the Spanish Association of Bovine Medicine Specialists.

TABLE OF CONTENTS

The importance of the dry period

The mammary gland of the dairy cow needs a period of rest at the end of lactation to prepare for the subsequent lactation; this is called the dry period and it usually lasts 42–60 days, although it is possible to cut it short.

It is a critical stage in the life of a cow, as a large number of intramammary infections (IMIs) can develop during this period and last until the next lactation; this in turn will affect the prevalence of clinical mastitis in the first 100 days of lactation, with an inevitable effect on milk production. The dry period is also important because IMIs from the previous lactation can be cured at this stage.

New IMIs can be prevented and the cure rate for existing IMIs can be increased. Treatment of all four quarters during drying-off is an essential part of any mastitis control programme.

Importance of the dry period

- Rest period for the udder
- Appearance of IMIs
- Effect on clinical mastitis in the following lactation

Objectives of the dry period

- Prevent IMIs
- Cure IMIs

Strategies

The rate of new infections during the dry period is usually higher than the rate of new infections during lactation. This information can be used to achieve the two objectives mentioned earlier: preventing new IMIs and curing any existing IMI.

- Increase the number of healthy quarters at calving by using antibiotic dry cow therapy (DCT). This increases the proportion of uninfected quarters by 8–14 %, depending on the author.
- Prevent IMIs by using internal teat sealants.

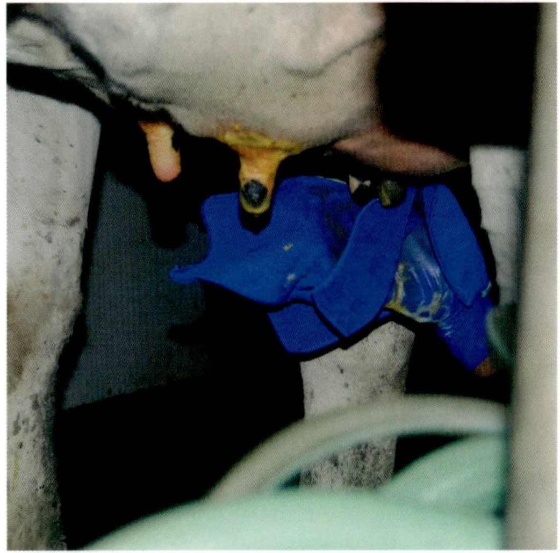

Figure 2. Cleaning and disinfecting the teats.

Financial impact

The most significant aspect of these infections is their effect on milk production in the following lactation. Quarters infected during the dry period subsequently produce 35 % less milk than healthy quarters, and quarters cured during the dry period subsequently produce 11 % less milk than quarters that have never been infected (Fig. 3).

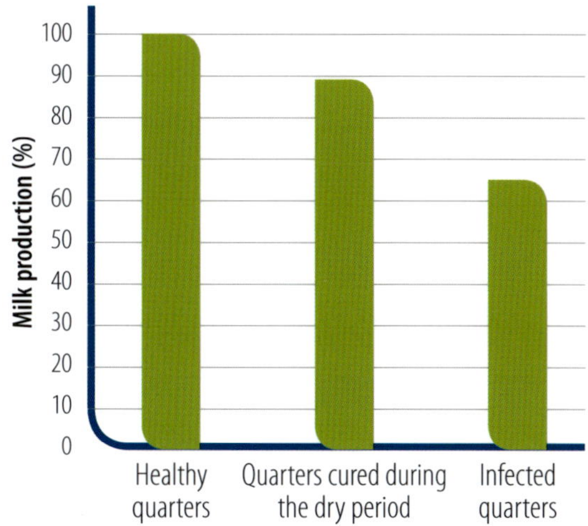

Figure 3. Milk production per quarter depending on their condition.

The financial impact of the dry period is very high, so management measures are required to reduce the prevalence of IMIs during this period and these should be included in an udder health programme. Implementation of strategies to achieve this requires knowledge of mammary gland physiology during drying-off, and in-depth understanding of epidemiology and the risk factors during the dry period.

The fundamental objective of the dry period is to achieve the lowest amount of IMIs to ensure a higher milk production in the subsequent lactation.

Strategies to control IMIs

- Implement a dry period.
- Use dry cow therapy.
- Protect the teat with internal/external teat sealants.
- Manage nutrition.
- Improve immunity.
- Manage the environment.
- Practice precalving milking.

Mammary involution

The physiology of the mammary gland during the dry period differs enormously from its physiology during lactation, for the simple reason that the primary and constant function of the mammary gland during lactation is to produce milk.

The mammary gland passes through three well-defined phases during the dry period:

- Active involution
- Steady state
- Colostrum or milk production

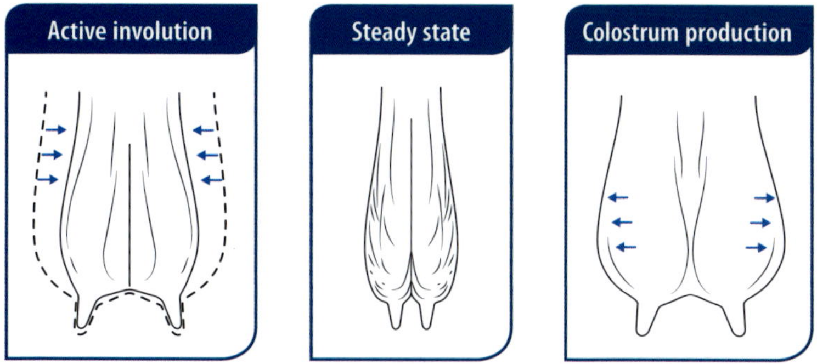

Figure 1. Diagram of udder morphology during the dry period.

Active involution phase

The active involution phase starts when milking ceases. The gland continues to produce milk, which accumulates in the udder and increases intramammary pressure. This increase in pressure largely depends on milk production; cows producing 10 litres per day will reach maximum intramammary pressure at 2–3 days after drying-off, and this will gradually decrease over the following 16 days, or even up to 30 days after drying-off.

In the first seven days of the dry period, the anatomy of the secretory epithelial cells (alveolar cells) and the composition of the mammary secretions change:

Changes in the secretory epithelial cells

Lysosomes participate actively in the phagocytosis of cell components, causing cellular autophagocytosis that reduces milk secretion dramatically. Programmed cell death, or apoptosis, takes place.

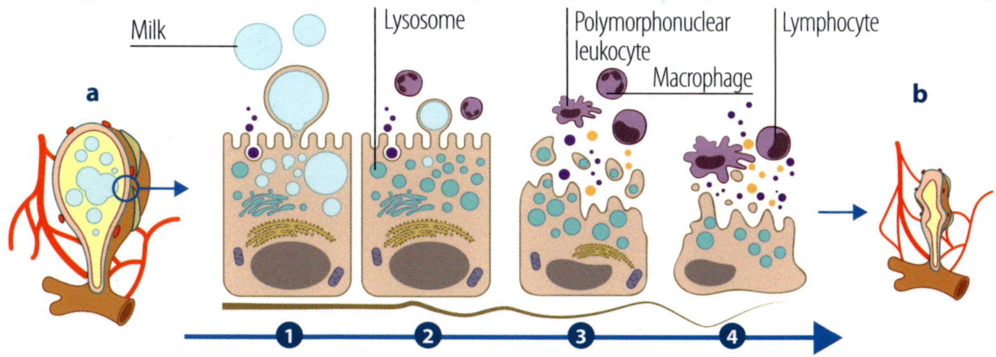

1. Epithelial cells produce milk in their cytoplasm and this is secreted into the lumen of the mammary alveoli, where it accumulates at the start of the dry period.
2. Lysosomes phagocytose cell components.
3. Death of the epithelial cells attracts neutrophils and macrophages that phagocytose the milk fat and protein release that occurs during cell death.
4. Macrophages, and lymphocytes which are more abundant in the final phases, efficiently phagocytose the cell remains, fat, and casein.

Figure 2. Process of involution of the milk-secreting epithelial cells. The alveolus in full milk production (a) undergoes changes that visibly reduce its volume (b).

Changes in the composition of mammary secretions

The changes that occur in the milk during the active involution phase affect levels of the following components:

- **Fat and proteins (casein, β-lactoglobulin and α-lactalbumin)** increase significantly from day 3 to day 7.
- **Lactose and citrate** decrease considerably.
- **Serum albumin** increases, due to increased permeability of the blood–milk barrier, although this increase never reaches the levels found in cases of acute mastitis during lactation.
- **Immunoglobulins (including IgG1, IgG2, IgA, and IgM)** increase, although much less than during the colostrum production phase.
- **Lactoferrin** increases very significantly, from 1.4 mg/ml on day 3 to 8.5 mg/ml on day 7, eventually becoming the most plentiful protein in the mammary gland during the dry period (20–30 mg/ml after 30 days).

Steady state phase

Once active involution is complete, the udder enters a phase where its volume and the number of secretory cells are at a minimum, and mammary secretion is negligible (only a few millilitres).

This phase lasts until hormones begin to change, indicating the start of the colostrum production phase.

Duration of this phase is very variable and can even be manipulated by nutritional measures aimed at minimising the dry period so that the cow can start a new lactation as soon as possible.

During this phase, lactose and citrate levels are below 5 mg/ml and 2 mg/ml respectively; the molar ratio of citrate to lactoferrin is maintained 100 times lower than during lactation, with immunoglobulin and lactoferrin levels remaining high.

Colostrum production phase

This phase starts two weeks before calving and is also known as lactogenesis. During this period, the gland prepares for colostrum production and storage. This phase is mediated by hormones. Udder volume grows in proportion to the number and activity of the secretory alveolar cells, and blood flow increases significantly, which can encourage udder oedema. Udder volume is greatest 1–3 days before calving.

The composition of the milk starts to change approximately five days before calving: fat, casein, and lactose levels increase; lactoferrin starts to decrease two weeks before calving, down to 2–3 mg/ml; and citrate levels increase significantly.

Colostrum confers passive immunity on the calf, because it is rich in immunoglobulins, especially IgG1.

Immunoglobulin levels start to rise 2–3 weeks before calving, peaking at 5–10 days before calving. The concentrations of IgG1, IgG2, IgA, and IgM in colostrum are approximately 60 mg/ml, 2.5 mg/ml, 4.5 mg/ml, and 6.0 mg/ml respectively.

Immunity in the mammary gland

Active involution phase

The active involution phase is critical to the development of IMIs and the reasons for the increased risk of infection can be divided into three categories, as follows:

1. **Anatomical factors:**
   - Increased intramammary pressure caused by accumulation of mammary secretions, to the extent where milk may even leak out.
   - Anatomical changes in the teat, which becomes wider and shorter, enabling bacteria to enter more easily.
   - The keratin plug begins to form.
2. **Hygiene factors:**
   - Routine disinfection practised during milking in the lactation period ceases.
   - The act of milking itself has the effect of flushing bacteria through the teat canal towards the exterior.

3. Immune factors:

- Milk composition does not change in the first three days, so there are hardly any defence factors at all.
- Immune defence cells, such as polymorphonuclear leukocytes (PMN) and macrophages, which should remove any potential bacteria, are occupied phagocytosing milk debris, such as fat and casein, and epithelial cells.
- Low lactoferrin levels in the first few days.
- Changes in diet and social group, where relationships with new animals have to be established, cause stress which, in turn, suppresses the immune system.

It is important that this phase is as short as possible to minimise the risk of mastitis. The shorter the active involution phase, the lower the risk of mastitis.

Mastitis risk factors during the dry period

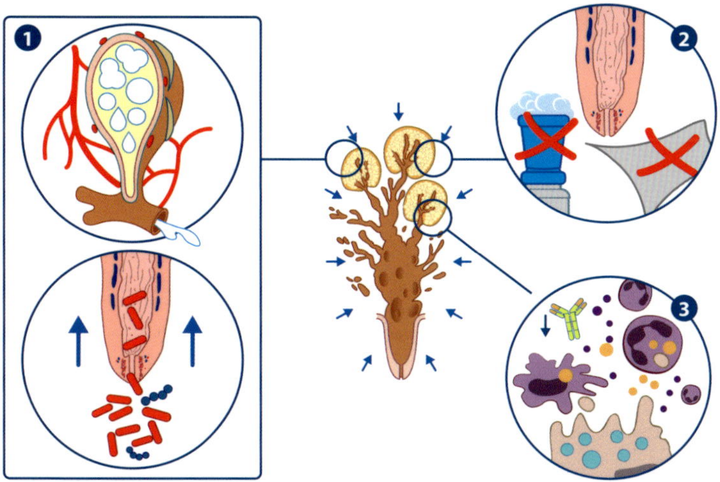

The changes that occur during the involution phase increase the risk of IMI.

1. **Milk accumulation:** causes leaking and changes in the teat before the keratin plug has formed.
2. Udder hygiene is reduced.
3. Period of immunosuppression: cells are occupied phagocytosing epithelial cells and milk residues, which can even act as nutrients for bacteria. Stress caused by nutritional changes also encourages this state.

Lactoferrin

This protein is involved in the udder's nonspecific defences during the dry period. It is produced in the lysosomes of the secretory cells and is also found in the granules of the PMNs. It acts as a mediator in the flow of PMNs, lymphocytes and macrophages, and therefore amplifies the immune response. It has a high binding affinity for iron, which is required for the survival of many mastitis-causing bacteria, such as coliforms (streptococci, for example, do not need much iron). As a result, it is an excellent bacteriostat in IMIs caused by bacteria such as coliforms and staphylococci.

When citrate is present, lactoferrin becomes less effective, as citrate is also an iron chelator and so competes for this element. The molar ratio of citrate to lactoferrin determines the degree of coliform growth in vitro.

The lower the citrate:lactoferrin molar ratio, the greater the inhibition of coliform growth.

Lactoferrin levels start to increase significantly from day 4 of the dry period.

Neutrophils, macrophages and lymphocytes

These cells phagocytose the remains of secretory cells, casein, and fat. Macrophages are the most important for this task; in fact, after seven days of involution, fat and casein levels decrease considerably, which indicates that the macrophages are working properly.

Polymorphonuclear leukocytes (neutrophils): the most numerous cells during the first week; levels later decrease.

Macrophages and lymphocytes: levels increase from days 14–30 of involution.

Steady state phase

During this phase, the udder is more resistant to IMIs caused by any kind of bacteria:

- There are large numbers of lymphocytes and macrophages; PMN numbers are lower.
- Lactoferrin levels are high.
- The keratin plug has formed in most cows.

The reduced capacity for phagocytosis by macrophages and PMNs, and low lactoferrin levels, are responsible for suppressing mammary gland immunity.

Colostrum production phase

The risk of infection increases in this phase due to immunosuppression, increased availability of milk components that continue to feed the bacteria, and the fact that many preparations that are used for intramammary dry cow therapy are inactive by the time this phase is reached.

Changes in udder defences can be summarised by the following factors:

Macrophages are present in the highest concentrations. Macrophages isolated from colostrum contain a large number of fat globules which, combined with the high casein levels that accumulate in the colostrum, reduce their capacity for phagocytosis.

Lymphocytes start to decrease two weeks before calving to levels 100-times lower than during the steady state phase. This reduction coincides with the fall in lactoferrin levels.

The molar ratio of citrate to lactoferrin increases, thus reducing the bacteriostatic properties of lactoferrin and increasing the likelihood that coliform bacteria will cause an IMI.

Suppression of the immune system (especially the cellular, or Th1, response) increases postpartum susceptibility to infectious diseases, such as mastitis and metritis.

There are two clearly defined periods of increased infection risk: the active involution and the colostrum production phases. The physiological, immunological, and anatomical changes that arise in these two periods pose the greatest risks.

In the active involution phase, epithelial cell activity decreases, but milk continues to accumulate in the udder, increasing intramammary pressure. The composition of the mammary secretion is characterised by lower levels of lactose, fat, casein, and citrate, higher pH, and higher levels of serum albumin, somatic cells, and lactoferrin.

During colostrum production, the secretory capacity of the epithelial cells increases to produce colostrum, and the blood–milk barrier becomes more permeable, which facilitates the passage of immunoglobulins (Ig), serum albumin, sodium and chloride to colostrum. Fat, protein, and lactose synthesis increase, which increases citrate and α-lactalbumin levels. Intramammary pressure increases during both periods, causing milk to leak out, which increases susceptibility to infection.

All of these physical, biochemical and hormonal changes that take place in the mammary gland during active involution and colostrum production increase susceptibility to new infections during the dry period (Fig. 1). All these factors mean microorganisms find the udder to be a welcoming environment, with a supply of nutrients and few defences that prevent them from becoming established.

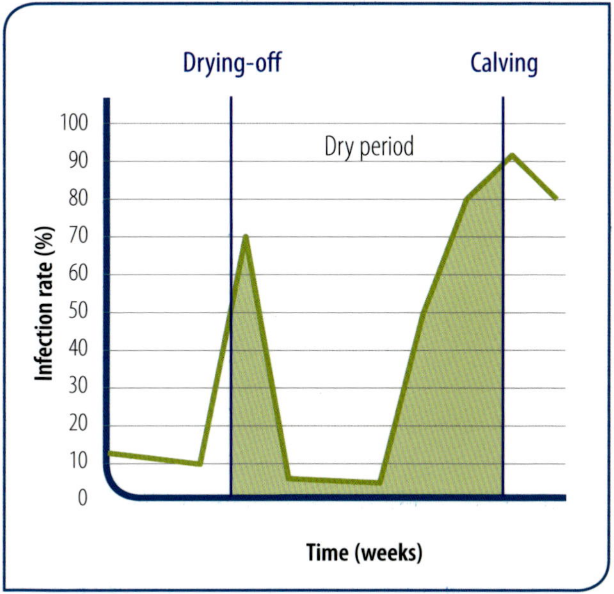

Figure 1. Mastitis risk. Note that the risk of infection is considerably lower during the dry period.

Factors affecting susceptibility

Three major groups of factors associated with the udder quarter, the cow, and the herd increase susceptibility to mastitis.

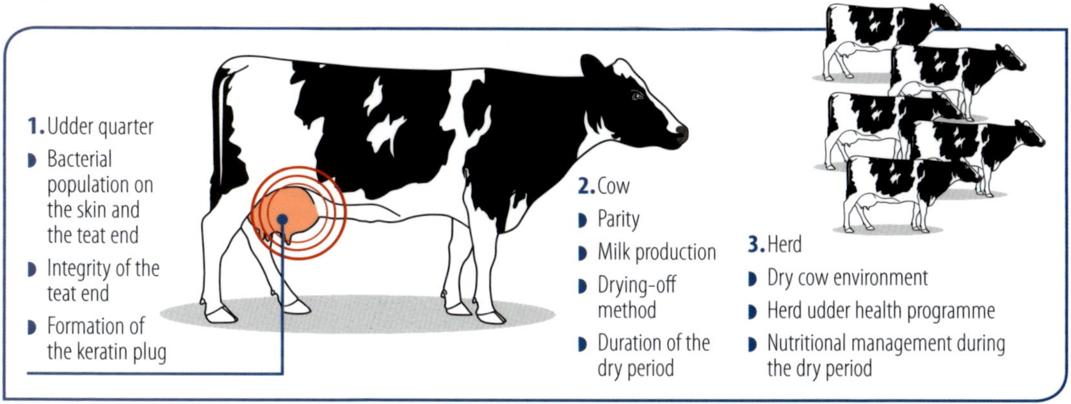

Figure 2. Factors associated with IMI development according to the environment in which they operate.

Udder quarter-related factors

Bacterial population on the skin and teat end

The bacterial population on the skin and teat end mainly depends on farm hygiene, which will determine the cleanliness of the cow and, therefore, the udder. Microorganisms such as staphylococci, streptococci, and gram-negative bacteria can be isolated from the cow's skin and teat end. As a general rule, more bacteria can be found at the start of the dry period, because the standard hygiene practices used during milking have stopped. Most of the bacteria found are coagulase-negative staphylococci, many of which cause infection during the dry period. This finding may indicate that these microorganisms protect against other potential infections, caused by, for example, streptococci and gram-negative bacteria. However, this theory has not been proven.

Microorganisms such as staphylococci, streptococci, and gram-negative bacteria can be isolated from the cow's skin and teat end.

Integrity of the teat end

There is a clear relationship between the teat end and the risk of infection. An increase in the surface area of the skin at the teat end, caused by hyperkeratosis, encourages bacteria to multiply, increasing the bacterial load and the likelihood of an infection developing.

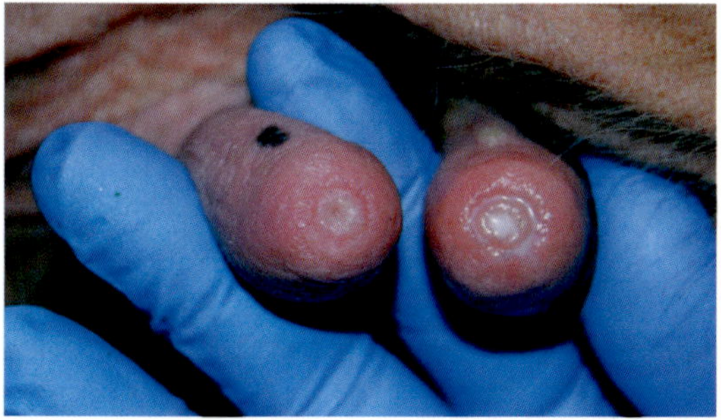

Figure 3. Healthy teats.

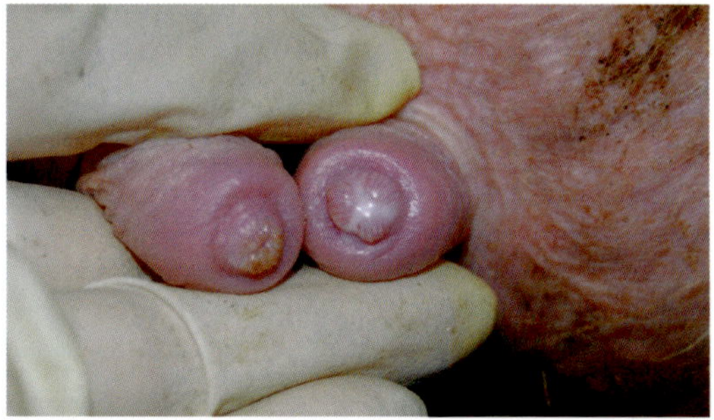

Figure 4. Teats with hyperkeratosis. Increased roughness increases the probability of an infection developing.

Formation of the keratin plug

The teat canal has two clear functions: to prevent milk from leaking out and to stop bacteria from entering the teat cistern. The keratin plug starts to form at the start of the dry period but the duration of the process until total closure happens varies depending on the cow. This has been confirmed by two classic studies (Fig. 5).

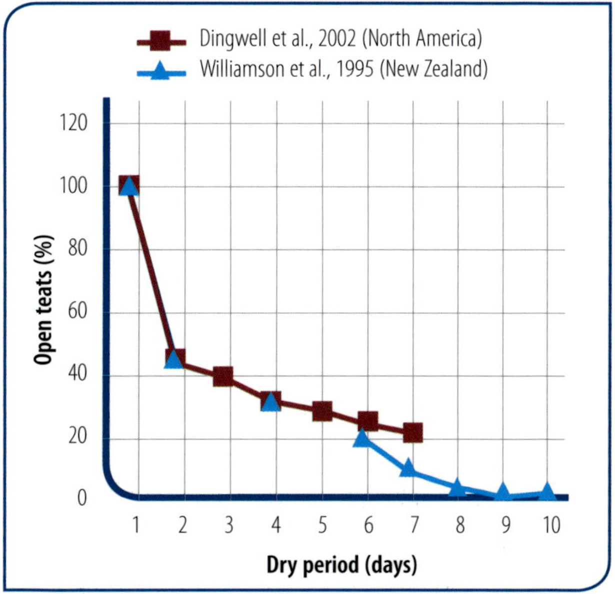

Figure 5. Development of the keratin plug in two studies.

Keratin is made up of fat from the milk, which gives it antibacterial properties. It is also a physical barrier to prevent microorganisms from entering. It is very important that the plug forms as quickly as possible to minimise infection.

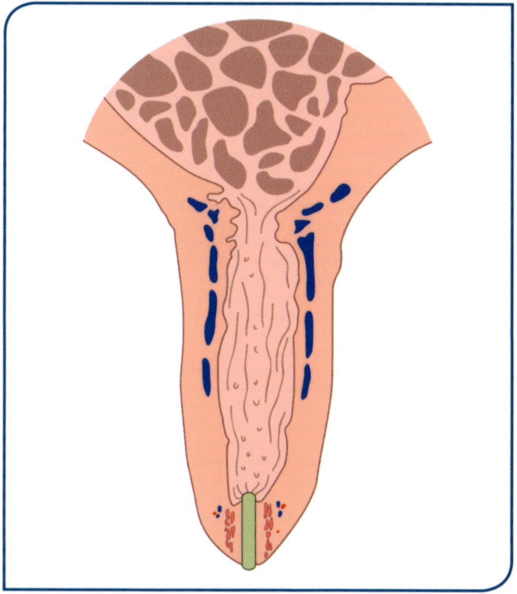

Figure 6. Diagram of the keratin plug.

Cow-related factors

Parity

As the cow gets older, the likelihood of acquiring a new IMI during the dry period increases. This occurs more frequently with infections caused by environmental streptococci, such as *Streptococcus uberis*, than with *Staphylococcus aureus* infections. This could be because active involution takes longer in mature adults than in younger animals.

It is advisable to dry cows off when they are producing less than 21 litres to ensure that the teat canal closes properly.

Milk production

The amount of milk still being produced by the cow at drying-off is a determining factor. Intramammary pressure has to be reduced for active involution to occur as quickly as possible. Lower pressure encourages the teats to close. The threshold established by the National Mastitis Council, based on studies carried out by Dingwell in 2002, is 21 litres. Above this, it is more likely that quarters remain open and infections occur, compared with cows that are dried off at a lower level of production.

Drying-off method

There are two methods of drying cows off: sudden cessation of milking (abrupt drying-off), or a phased reduction in milk production (gradual drying-off).

Abrupt drying-off: Following a normal milking regime, the cow is transferred directly to the dry cow group. The disadvantage of this drying-off method is the increase in intramammary pressure, and the associated increased risk of milk leaking out, with discomfort and pain.

Gradual drying-off: Milk production is reduced by milking at alternate sessions, or controlling the diet during the preceding days. Gradual drying-off by reducing feed intake causes stress and hunger, and suppresses the immune system. If the frequency of milking is reduced, active involution is prolonged and there is a greater risk of IMI.

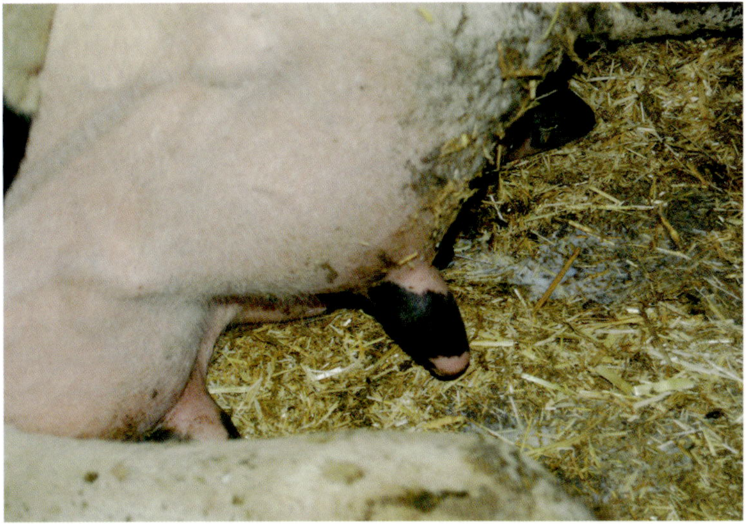

Figure 7. Increased pressure causes milk to leak out, encouraging IMIs.

Duration of the dry period

The dry period usually lasts 42–60 days. Cutting this period short helps maintain milk production on the farm at the time, but the cow's production will be reduced in the following lactation. This does not increase the likelihood of acquiring new infections, but any infections that are already present are less likely to be cured.

The cow's age and milk production are important factors in determining the occurrence of IMIs. However, management at drying-off and the duration of the dry period also determine udder health in the dry cow.

Herd-related factors

Dry cow environment

The more the dry cow is exposed to the bacteria that cause mastitis, the greater the probability that infection will occur. Management of the cow's bedding is a crucial factor. Herds housed on farms with poor hygiene management and environmental conditions develop more infections.

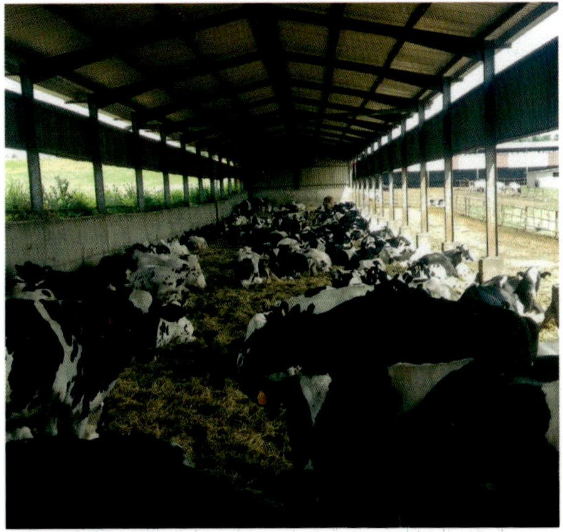

Figure 8. Dry cows housed in a suitable environment are less likely to develop an IMI.

Udder health programmes

Herds that implement measures to prevent mastitis at every level, including the comfort of the cow in the dry period and during lactation, an appropriate milking routine, correctly functioning milking equipment, etc., will be less likely to develop infections during the dry period.

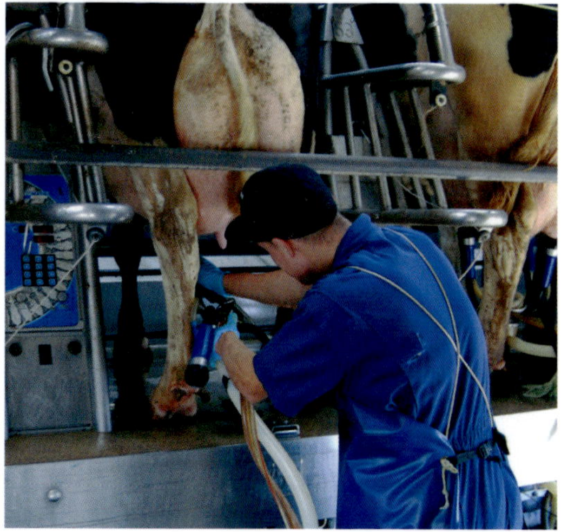

Figure 9. Correct hygiene management during milking also prevents IMIs.

Nutritional management during the dry period

Immune function plays an important role in determining udder health in the dry cow, and this is fundamentally affected by nutrition. Reducing dry matter intake causes a negative energy balance which increases the risk of developing mastitis and other disorders, such as ketosis, retained placenta and displaced abomasum. This can occur when the diet is suddenly changed when the cow is dried off; the reduced ration increases levels of non-esterified fatty acids that directly affect neutrophil function. Calcium deficiency also often results from this sudden change and increases the occurrence of IMIs, and vitamin and mineral levels affect the cow's immune function.

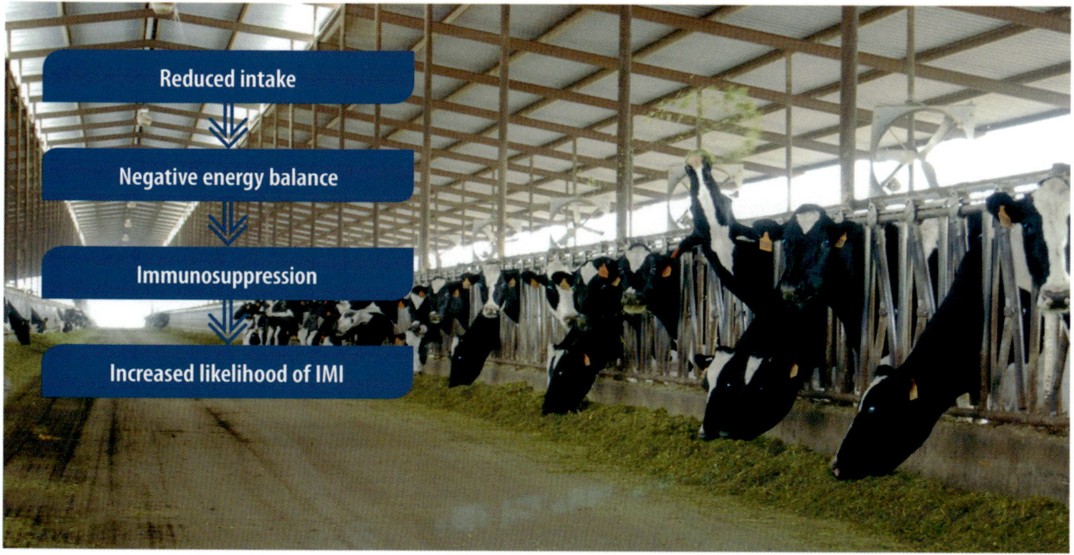
Reduced intake
Negative energy balance
Immunosuppression
Increased likelihood of IMI

Figure 10. Reduced feed intake during the dry period can be detrimental to the immune status of the cow.

Table 1. Factors that increase the risk of IMI at drying-off.

Udder	Bacterial population	Udder cleanliness
	Teat integrity	Hyperkeratosis
	Keratin plug	Late formation
Cow	Parity	Older cows
	High milk production	Increased intramammary pressure
	Drying-off method	Abrupt Gradual
	Duration of the dry period	Short
Herd	Environment	Poor on-farm hygiene
	Prevention	Ineffective or nonexistent preventive measures
	Nutrition	Poor management, sudden changes

Welfare of the dairy cow

Animal welfare is defined as the absence of suffering. Five conditions must be met in order for this to be possible in animal production:

1. Adequate food and water supply.
2. Comfortable ambient temperature.
3. Facilities suited to the characteristics of the animal.
4. Ability to display natural behaviour.
5. Absence of stress.

However, the cow undergoes a series of changes caused by drying-off that alter her welfare status and cause a situation of stress:

- Cessation of milking.
- Dietary changes.
- Housing changes.

Two stressful periods can therefore be differentiated with respect to dry cow welfare: the actual moment when cows are dried off and the few following days, and the dry period itself.

Consequences of drying-off

When a cow is dried off, particularly if drying-off is abrupt, the cow suffers pain and discomfort, mainly due to an accumulation of milk that increases intramammary pressure. This milk retention can lead to tissue damage that also causes pain. In addition, rations or water intake may also be restricted.

These actions all inevitably reduce the animal's welfare and cause stress.

In addition to all these factors, the cow may also be suffering from mastitis, considered to be one of the most painful conditions for a dairy cow.

Causes of stress at drying-off

- Pain caused by milk accumulation
- Pain caused by tissue damage
- Pain caused by IMIs
- Restricted diet or water

The cow at drying-off suffers pain, stress and frustration caused by increased intramammary pressure, and nutritional and management changes.

Stress caused by pain

All animals feel pain, which is defined as a disagreeable sensory and emotional experience associated with real or potential tissue damage. However, manifestation of this pain depends on the animal involved. It is usually difficult to detect pain in a dairy cow because of their placid nature and limited vocalisation in unpleasant situations.

About 10 to 20 % of dry cows suffer pain as a result of intramammary pressure caused by the accumulation of milk, and approximately 6 % suffer very severe pain.

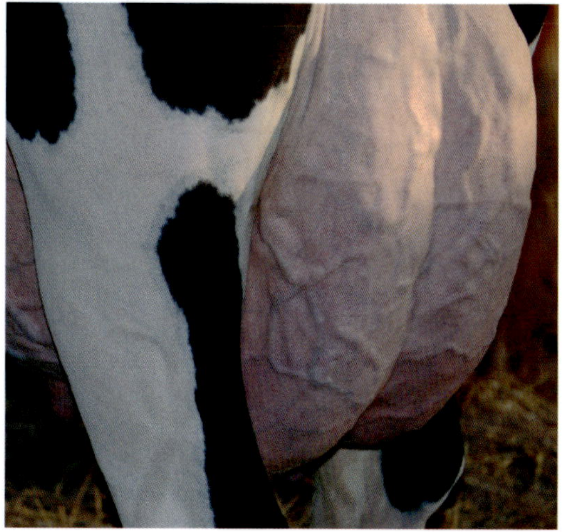

Figure 1. The appearance of this udder indicates milk retention and will give an idea of the cow's level of discomfort or pain.

Measuring pain

The severity of pain can be measured objectively, using pain indicators that are usually related to behavioural changes. Other indicators are physiological, associated with dry matter intake and reduced rumen motility (reduced digestion).

Pain indicators

Behavioural indicators are the most important in practice, as they are the easiest way to allow pain to be assessed and quantified. In order to use these indicators, it is essential to be familiar with cow behaviour in general at drying-off and during the dry period.

Some behavioural indicators will increase and others, conversely, will reduce:

- Longer periods standing up (lying down increases the pain due to pressure on the udder).
- Hocks more straddled (contact between udder and legs increases the pain).
- Head movements increase. The cow shakes her head and ears more often.
- Scratching behaviour increases.
- There may be more kicking.
- Pain on palpation.

There may be increased vocalisation when intramammary pressure is high. Some authors suggest that this phenomenon occurs when there is more than 25 kg of milk in the udder.

Another method of assessing pain is to observe the length of time a dry cow spends resting. It seems that dry cows with high intramammary pressure (>25 kg of milk) spend longer standing up.

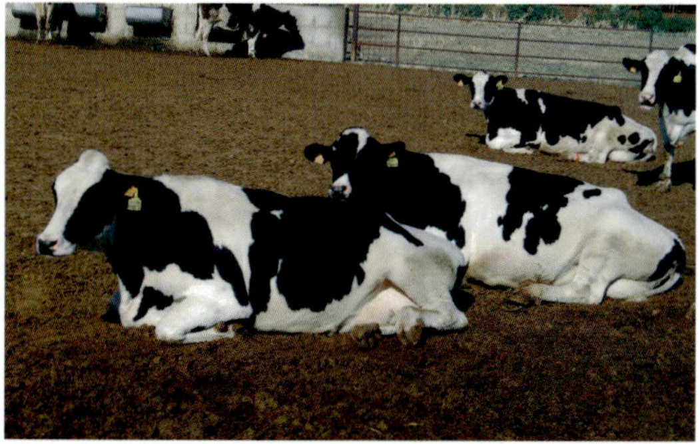

Figure 2. Dry cows resting.

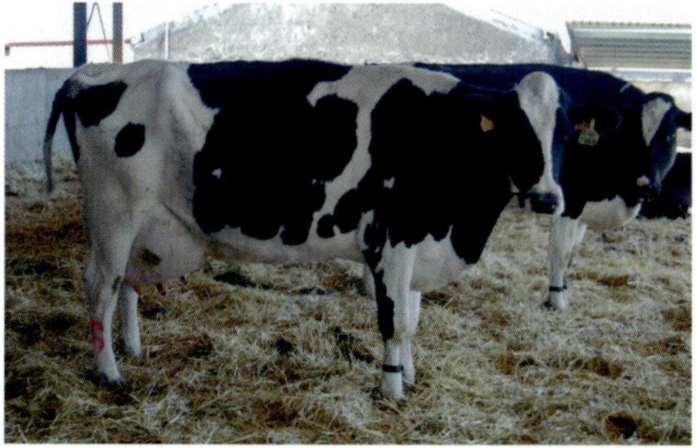

Figure 3. Cows standing up can suggest udder pain and a possible IMI.

Pain on palpation

A reaction to palpation is also useful to assess the pain suffered by the cow.

Dry cows with mastitis exhibit allodynia, so stimuli such as palpation that would not normally cause pain or any reaction from the cow become painful stimuli that trigger a reaction as a result of the mastitis. Three levels of allodynia have been established in function of the intensity of this reaction:

- **Level 0:** No reaction to palpation.
- **Level 1 or mild:** Slight reaction (movement of the feet, change of posture, signs of nervousness such as slight movements of the tail or head).
- **Level 2 or moderate:** Obvious reaction (raises a hind leg, abrupt movements of the tail and/or head).
- **Level 3 or severe:** The cow reacts violently in total rejection of palpation (kicks, moves abruptly).

In addition to observation and palpation, the pain suffered by the cow can also be monitored by the use of pedometers that measure cow activity, and algorithms can be used to determine intramammary pressure.

Stress caused by nutritional changes

Drying a cow off involves restricting the diet or water. To facilitate drying-off, dry matter intake is reduced by feeding a diet containing less energy, and increasing the amount of less palatable forage. These changes make the cow hungry, which is detrimental to her welfare. The cow reacts to this state of hunger by increasing vocalisation, which is considered to be a behavioural indicator of stress.

Ultimately, when feed is restricted, stress increases levels of cortisol and some glucocorticoid metabolites, such as 11,17-dioxoandrostane, in the blood, and these can be detected in the faeces of cows that have been dried off and are suffering from high intramammary pressure.

The glucocorticoid metabolite 11,17-dioxoandrostane is a physiological indicator of stress that can be detected in animal faeces.

Stress caused by heat

Cow welfare during the dry period tends to be overlooked, mainly because the cow is not producing milk. This is a serious mistake, as dry cows can suffer maximum stress during the transition or prepartum period, a truly critical moment in the cycle due to its effect on the subsequent lactation.

During the dry period, the cow is mainly affected by the changes in dietary reductions and pain from milk retention as described above, which may or may not be associated with an IMI. However, heat will particularly affect the dry cow and may be the main cause of stress with very significant repercussions on milk production.

Consequences of heat stress:

- Changes in liver metabolism → disruption of cellular immunity (causing immunosuppression) → predisposition to intramammary infections.
- Reduced dry matter consumption → reduced proliferation of mammary epithelial cells (not affecting the mammary stroma) → reduced production in the following lactation.
- Reduced feed consumption → the cow loses weight→ shorter gestation period with a shorter dry period → calf birth weight is lower.

Managing ambient temperature reduces heat stress.

Cows housed on farms where high ambient temperatures are controlled by the use of appliances such as fans and sprinklers have a lower rectal temperature and lower respiration rate, as a result of an optimal ambient temperature.

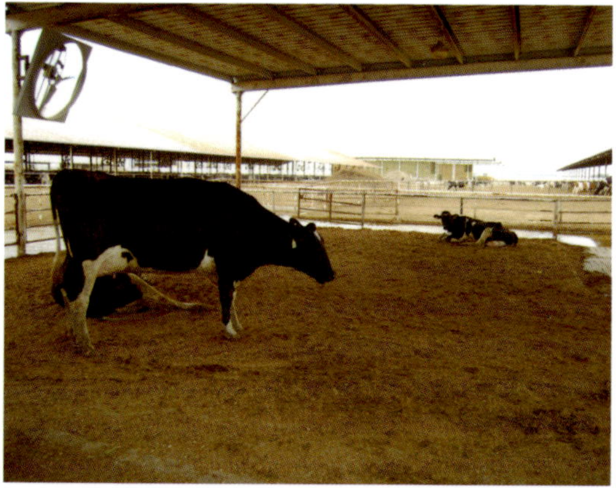

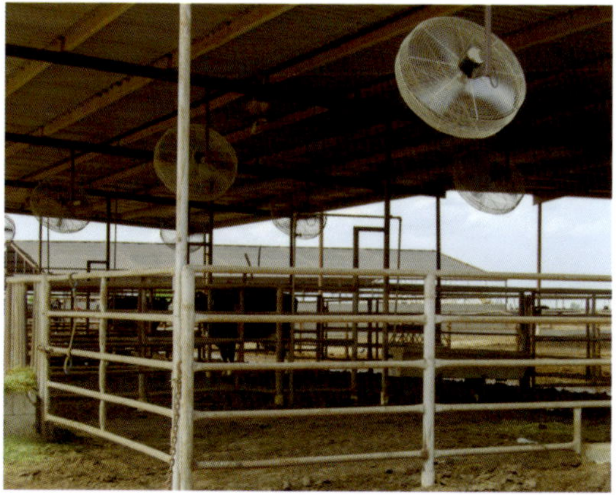

Figures 4 and 5. Using fans to manage high ambient temperature reduces heat stress in dry cows.

Heat stress causes additional energy loss through panting and sweating, and reduced intake, which reduces milk production during the following lactation.

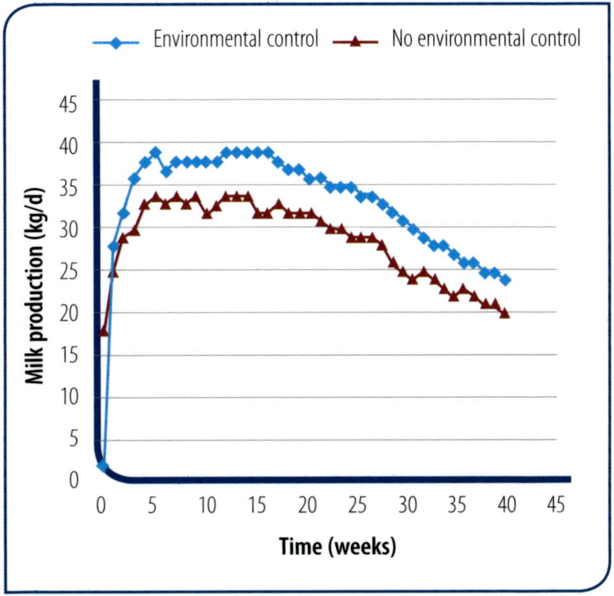

Figure 6. Effect of heat stress in dry cows on production during the following lactation. The blue line represents production by cows in environments where high temperatures are controlled by fans; the red line represents production by cows suffering from heat stress (no ventilation). Data adapted from Tao et al., 2011.

The purpose of the dry period is to combat any new IMI that may occur during this time, and to prevent any that do occur from causing various problems in the next lactation. These include new cases of clinical mastitis, reduced milk production, increased possibility of infecting other animals and, of course, poor milk quality, mainly due to an increased somatic cell count (SCC).

Objectives of the dry period: to prevent new infections and cure existing ones.

This period is also used to cure existing infections. Different strategies can be used by the veterinary practitioner to achieve these objectives, depending on how the farm operates:

- Drying-off methods
- Dry cow therapy. Selective dry cow therapy
- Teat protection
- Nutritional management
- Immune system support
- Environmental control
- Precalving milking
- Epidemiological control during the dry period

Drying-off methods

The drying-off method is understood to mean the procedure used to dry off, or stop milk production in, a lactating cow.

There are two methods for drying cows off: abrupt (or sudden) and gradual. Abrupt drying-off consists of a sudden cessation of milking on a date established by the farm in relation to the predicted calving date. The gradual method consists of intermittent milking, or reducing milking frequency, in the last week of milking, and the main objective is to reduce milk production. Other authors include in gradual drying-off a method that consists of an abrupt cessation of milking coupled with simultaneous dietary changes or restriction to reduce milk production. Dietary restriction can be used in both methods.

Water intake should never be restricted during the drying-off process.

The biggest problem in the drying-off period is milk production, as the risk of infection is greater at higher levels of production. This factor is more obvious in abrupt drying-off, as milk retention is greater.

Gradual drying-off involves reducing milk production and the volume of milk retained, and it is associated with less milk leakage by squirting or dripping, reduced IMIs at calving and, therefore, improved udder health. The disadvantage of this method is its management, which is complicated in practice.

Many studies have been conducted to discover the best drying-off method, and results have varied: the first studies demonstrated that gradual drying-off reduces the amount of IMIs; other more recent studies have shown that cows dried off gradually give less milk. It has also been demonstrated that multiparous cows that are dried off gradually and have an IMI at drying-off, and primiparous cows that are dried off abruptly with milk leakage, are at greatest risk of infection at calving. It has recently been concluded that the occurrence of new infections is affected more by the presence of pathogens at drying-off than by milk production at drying-off.

The existence of pathogens at drying-off affects the occurrence of IMIs more than the volume of milk produced.

Advantages and disadvantages of drying-off methods

Both types of drying-off have their advantages and disadvantages.

Gradual drying-off: In general, milk leakage, and therefore the risk of IMI at calving, decreases with reduced production. Disadvantages: milking at alternate sessions increases the duration of the active involution phase and its associated risks. This method is normally linked to dietary changes, which continue through the drying-off period, potentially causing stress and hunger, and suppressing the immune system. Another great disadvantage is the difficulty of implementing this method on large farms.

Abrupt drying-off: Easier management, as all the cows on the farm are milked with the same frequency. The disadvantage is that milk leakage by squirting or dripping can increase, raising the probability of infection at calving. This method of drying cows off increases intramammary pressure which is likely to cause more discomfort and pain.

Despite the disadvantages of this method, abrupt drying-off is used on most dairy farms. In fact, 90 % of herds that are milk recorded in the United States are dried off abruptly.

In conclusion, the ideal situation is thought to be to dry cows off when they are producing less than 21 kg of milk, thus preventing intramammary pressure from increasing and reducing milk leakage. This can be achieved with an abrupt drying-off, with a slight dietary change where possible. It would be very useful to use different techniques that would enable milk production to be reduced without causing stress to the animal.

Ideally, cows should be dried off when they are producing less than 21 kg of milk.

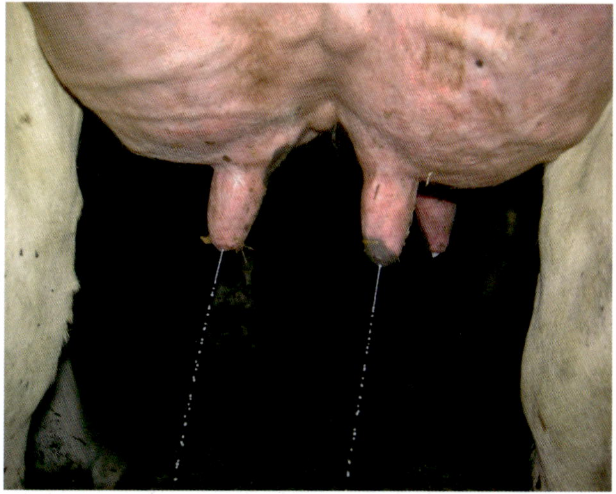

Figure 1. Increased intramammary pressure can cause milk leakage with the associated risk of IMI.

Dry cow therapy

Intramammary therapy

Dry cow therapy consists of administering an antibiotic through the teat canal using a nozzle. The aim is to eliminate existing infections and prevent any new ones from developing. The products used should reach high concentrations in the mammary parenchyma and be long-acting to prolong their effect.

Any antimicrobials used should reach high concentrations in the mammary parenchyma and be long-acting.

This treatment (initially penicillin) was originally used to combat major contagious pathogens, such as *Staphylococcus aureus* and *Streptococcus agalactiae*. The spectrum was subsequently widened to include gram-negative bacteria, so amoxicillin and cephalosporins started to be used. Penethamate, cloxacillin, and cephalosporins are the products most commonly used today.

Careful administration of intramammary therapy

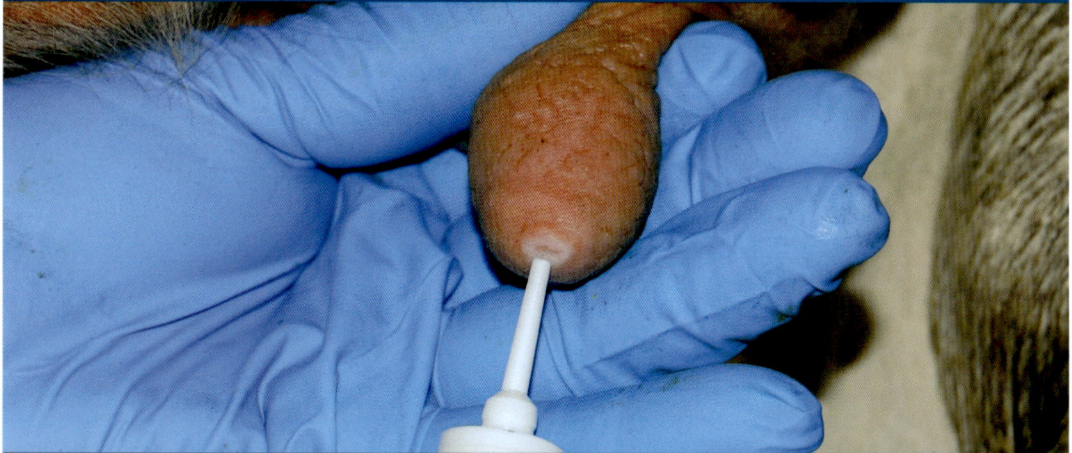

Hygiene measures should be adopted when using an intramammary nozzle, such as only introducing the tip of the cannula to prevent damage to the internal mucosa of the teat cistern.

Determining pathogen susceptibility is a factor that must be considered to achieve maximum treatment efficacy.

Table 1. Spectrum of activity of the antibiotics commonly used to treat dry cows in the United Kingdom (adapted from Bradley and Green, 2007).

	Gram-positive bacteria	β-Lactamase-producing *S. aureus*	Gram-negative bacteria
Penicillins/penethamate	+++	-	-
Ampicillin	++	-	+
Cloxacillin/nafcillin	+++	+++	-
Cephalonium	++	++	++
Cefquinome	++	++	++
Dihydrostreptomycin	+	++	+++
Framycetin/neomycin	++	++	+++

It is essential to understand the epidemiology of infections found on the farm in order to choose the most effective antimicrobial treatment.

According to studies conducted by Soback et al. in 1992, the efficacy of an antimicrobial therapy depends on the following factors:

- An adequate concentration of antibiotic is maintained at the infection site for an adequate period.
- Susceptibility of the bacteria to the antibiotic.
- Antibiotic pharmacodynamics.
- Dose and form of administration.
- Timing of antibiotic therapy (in this case, while drying off the udder).
- Presence of intracellular bacteria (*Staphylococcus aureus* or *Streptococcus uberis*), which can impede antibiotic access.
- Reinfection. This occurs when a small number of bacteria survive the antibiotic, and the udder's defence mechanisms cannot eliminate them completely.

Systemic therapy

The aim of this type of treatment is to increase the cure rate. Penethamate, quinolones, and macrolides may be used, again depending on the aetiology of the infection. In this case, it is necessary to ascertain whether an infection is present when the cow is dried off, and it is useful to take a sample of milk at drying-off and test it to discover what micro-organisms are present.

This type of treatment tends to be used on farms where only environmental microorganisms are detected, and where attempts are made to cure as many cows as possible with an infection at drying-off.

Procedure

- Combine samples of milk from all four quarters at drying-off.
- If a major pathogen, such as *Streptococcus uberis*, *Corynebacterium* spp., *Streptococcus dysgalactiae*, *Trueperella pyogenes*, or enterobacteria, such as *Escherichia coli*, are detected, treat the cow.
- Treatment of choice: quinolone for gram-negative bacteria and penethamate for gram-positive bacteria.
- Confirm efficacy: combine samples of milk from all four quarters in the first week after calving.

The author has observed that very good cure rates can be achieved: 75 % for gram-positive and 80 % for gram-negative bacteria.

Blanket therapy

This consists of treating 100 % of the cows at drying-off. This method has been practised for over 60 years, and farmers are familiar with it.

However, the procedure has been called into question recently, as it involves a high level of antibiotic use in production animals when reasonable antibiotic use is currently the aim. Most of the antibiotics used in dairy cattle are aimed at udder health, and most of these are used as dry cow therapy.

This is why the practice known as selective dry cow therapy is being promoted.

Selective dry cow therapy

This is already being used in some countries to reduce antibiotic use and antimicrobial resistance. As much information as possible should be gathered about herd udder health in order to adopt this strategy during drying-off:

1. Bulk milk SCC
2. Individual SCC
3. Microbiological analysis of the milk at drying-off
4. Record of clinical mastitis cases

All of these data provide precise information on herd epidemiology, and therefore the herd's udder health. It is then possible to decide whether the farm is high risk or low risk.

- **High-risk farms:** bulk milk cell counts over 250,000 cells/ml and/or presence of contagious microorganisms, such as *Streptococcus agalactiae* or *Staphylococcus aureus*.
- **Low-risk farms:** bulk milk cell counts under 250,000 cells/ml and no contagious microorganisms.

Selective dry cow therapy is only suitable for low-risk farms.

Guidelines for the use of selective dry cow therapy

- All cows are usually treated with an internal teat sealant.
- If the cow's SCC has been over 200,000 cells/ml at any of her last three readings, dry cow therapy should be administered.
- If the cow has had a case of clinical mastitis in the previous three months, dry cow therapy should be administered.

This strategy cannot be employed on all farms, as not all farms are part of an official milk-recording programme, so sampling the milk for microbial culture at drying-off is very useful.

In general, selective dry cow therapy affects the farm's quality results as follows:

- Farm SCCs increase.
- The number of cases of clinical mastitis that arise during the first 100 days of lactation increases.

The dairy sector has to accept that reducing antibiotic use can reduce milk quality.

Teat protection

It is essential to seal the teat to prevent microorganisms from entering. The keratin plug forms naturally to prevent new infections. It takes an average of two weeks to form, but it is a well-known fact that it may never form in many cows. To compensate for this, it is a good idea to apply a teat sealant which forms a physical barrier that prevents micro-organisms from entering.

These products are used to reduce new infections, mainly caused by environmental pathogens.

Teats can be sealed in two ways, which give the type of sealant their name:

- Internal sealants
- External sealants

Internal sealants

The aim of the internal sealant is to act as a physical barrier to reduce the bacteria that enter through the teat canal, especially environmental bacteria such as streptococci and enterobacteria. Sealants persist through the whole dry period, sometimes for as long as 100 days. Their formulation includes bismuth subnitrate in a paraffin base.

The sealant can be applied in combination with a dry cow therapy, or alone: when applied in combination, the antimicrobial should be administered first, then the sealant.

The application process is critical: disinfect the teat end, constrict the top of the teat and introduce the sealant nozzle. This method ensures that most of the sealant remains in the teat cistern. When the cow calves, the sealant is usually removed in the first streams of milk, indicating that it has behaved correctly, although sometimes it can appear during a subsequent milking.

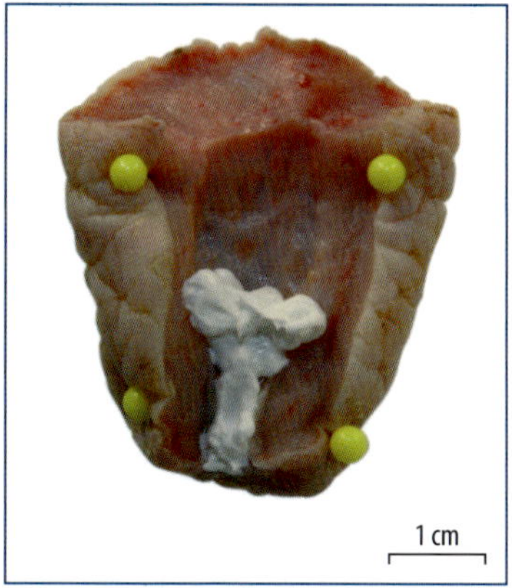

Figure 2. Once the sealant has been inserted into the teat canal, it should remain in the teat cistern. Image courtesy of Peter Edmondson.

Efficacy of internal sealants

Many studies have been carried out to confirm the efficacy of internal sealants and the results obtained in the various circumstances proposed prove that there is hardly any difference between infection rates in animals treated with antibiotics only, and those treated with an antibiotic and a sealant. However, there is a great difference between animals administered an internal sealant and those with no sealant. In fact, a recent (unpublished) study carried out by the author demonstrated the efficacy of internal sealants, with a rate of new infections in freshly calved cows of 10.4 % on farms that used internal sealants, compared to 22 % on farm that did not use the sealant.

In the author's opinion, farms that use internal sealants have lower rates of new infections in freshly calved cows. In the author's experience, using an internal sealant usually results in 50 % fewer new infections.

Farms that use internal sealants have 50 % fewer new infections.

External sealants

External sealants form an external physical barrier around the teat to prevent bacteria from entering the teat cistern. Their formulation includes substances such as latex and other types of polymer. These products are usually applied twice during the dry period (at the critical stages of drying-off and precalving) because they only function for up to ten days, although Hemling et al. (2000) found that the average duration was actually seven days.

Studies carried out over the last decade have demonstrated the efficacy of external sealants applied at drying-off and ten days before calving, reducing IMIs in freshly calved cows by 47 % and in heifers by 19 % (Timms, 2001).

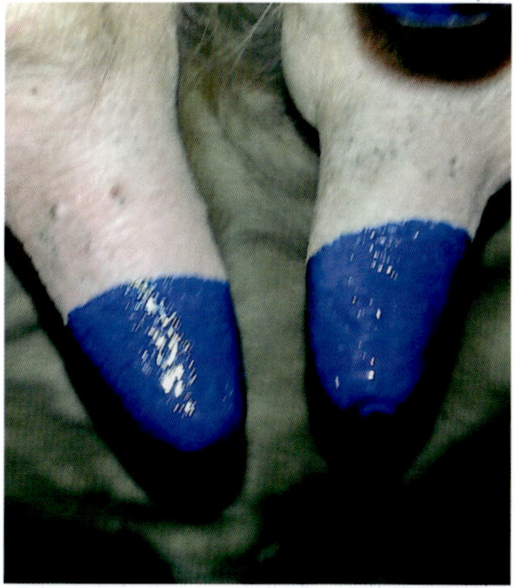

Figure 3. External sealant.

Nutritional management

The immune system needs appropriate nutrition to function well. The fact that cows suffer a certain degree of physiological stress due to dietary changes, changes in animal groupings, and calving must be taken into account. These changes all reduce dry matter intake, which disrupts the immune system and, therefore, udder health and milk production.

Effect of reduced dry matter intake

- Levels of nonesterified fatty acids (NEFAs) in the blood increase, compromising immune function and increasing the risk of mastitis. Blood testing is very useful to detect NEFAs and confirm/rule out problems with the diet.

- The potential for subclinical ketosis increases. This metabolic disease also has an adverse effect on immune function and, therefore, on the occurrence of mastitis.
- The risk of hypocalcaemia increases. It is important to prevent this from occurring during the precalving period, as calcium affects reproductive efficiency, milk production and the cow's general health postpartum, including the incidence of IMIs.

Levels of vitamins A and E, selenium, zinc, and copper also affect the immune function, particularly the functioning of epithelial cells.

As a result, dry cows must ingest enough energy during the dry period to ensure that they remain in positive energy balance and their immune system is not disrupted.

Key points for nutrition during the dry period

- **Ensure dry matter intake is maintained.**
- **Prevent/control metabolic diseases.**
- **Provide vitamin and mineral supplements.**

The transition phase is crucial, and particular attention must be paid to:

- Ration formulation, palatability and the condition of the feeder.
- Potential metabolic diseases. Early diagnosis enables rapid action to correct nutrition, maintaining good immune system functioning and preventing clinical and subclinical mastitis.
- Udder oedema. Prevention reduces the risk of clinical mastitis at calving. Oedema tends to be associated with high-salt diets, so prevention includes avoiding an excess of salt precalving, and using anionic salts in the diet. Exercise can help prevent udder oedema. In severe cases, the cow will have to be milked before calving.

Prepartum udder oedema

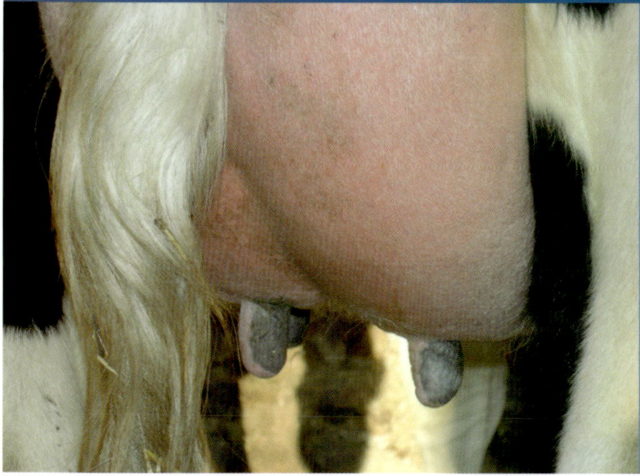

Udder oedema is an excessive accumulation of lymphatic fluid in the interstitial space. It tends to start a few days before calving and continues for at least three weeks after calving. It tends to be more common in adult cows than in heifers. The cause is unknown, although it is related to genetics, circulatory problems and nutrition (Lema et al., 1992).

Immune system support

The cow's immune system is suppressed in the transition period due to all the changes occurring at this time and the cow is at greatest risk during this period from new infections that can develop into clinical mastitis in the first 100 days of lactation.

Ensuring good function of the immune system is therefore the best way to prevent new infections and reduce the frequency, duration, and severity of any clinical mastitis that does occur.

Vaccinating against mastitis is a key part of on-farm mastitis control programmes.

The cow's immune defences and resistance to infection by gram-negative bacteria can be boosted by vaccination. These vaccines contain an antigen called "core" or "J5", which is common to all coliform bacteria. Results from field trials on the efficacy of this vaccine have been good, with a significantly lower incidence of clinical mastitis (González, 1989; Cullor, 1991; and Hogan, 1992).

Experimental studies with the core antigen have demonstrated that these vaccines do not reduce the number of new infections caused by coliform bacteria, but they do reduce the incidence and severity of clinical mastitis caused by these microorganisms. Development of these vaccines represents a significant advance in the transfer of active immunity, and they should be used as part of the farm's mastitis control programme, to reduce clinical mastitis caused by coliform bacteria.

Vaccines do not reduce new infections by coliform bacteria, but they do reduce the incidence and severity of mastitis caused by these bacteria.

Environmental control

Most microorganisms that cause IMIs are found in the environment, so dry cow housing should be kept in an extremely clean and hygienic condition. Environmental conditions also affect cow comfort, minimising stress and improving the immune response.

The best dry cow facilities are clean, dry, and comfortable. These are essential prerequisites. Options for dry cow accommodation are cubicles, straw yards or compost bedded pack barns.

It is also important to control vectors, such as flies, which can transmit microorganisms that cause mastitis.

Pasture

If dry cows are kept at pasture, the grazing must be well drained and cows must have easy access to feeders and drinkers, and to shelter. Dry cow housing is usually a combination of loose housing with access to a yard.

Dry cow pasture must be well drained and cows must have access to feeders and drinkers.

Cubicle housing

The cubicles should be a little wider than milking cow cubicles (approximately 125 cm wide) to ensure that the cow can lie down and get up easily. The most popular bedding is sand, as it offers better standards of hygiene and comfort. It is also less attractive to microorganisms. Dung should be removed from the bedding twice a day, and clean bedding added to the rear of the cubicle. Feeder passages and loafing areas should be cleaned out at least twice a day, to ensure that they are always clean and dry.

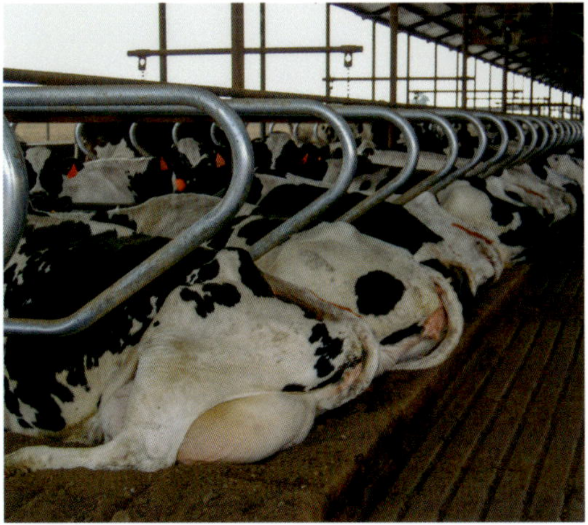

Figure 4. The cubicle should be well designed and have sufficient bedding: sand is the most appropriate.

Straw yard housing

This system is still in use and it is very common to see it in the calving area. This type of housing should meet the following requirements:

- Space per cow. Ideally more than 10 m^2/cow for the cow to be comfortable.
- Cleanliness and hygiene. Bedding should be maintained in the best condition possible:
  - 7–8 kg per cow per day.
  - Disinfect the bedding with substances such as calcium superphosphate twice a week.
- The loafing area should be cleaned out at least three times a week, depending on the time of year.

Applying these measures prevents the resting area from becoming too contaminated. Manure should never be allowed to accumulate, and there should not be any puddles, etc., as these are the areas where the most mastitis-causing microorganisms can be found.

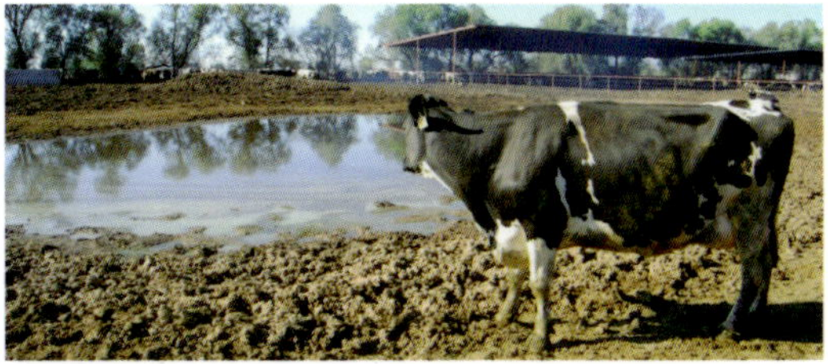

Figure 5. Poor facilities are a source of bacteria that cause mastitis.

Infections can occur during the dry period in this type of facility, mainly caused by environmental streptococci and coliform bacteria, as bedding material is an excellent substrate for these micro-organisms and it is very difficult to keep bedding in a good condition. Calving areas are a different scenario: an all-in/all-out system should be used, and the cow should remain in the calving area for a maximum of 24 hours.

It is important to control the vectors that transmit mastitis during the dry period.

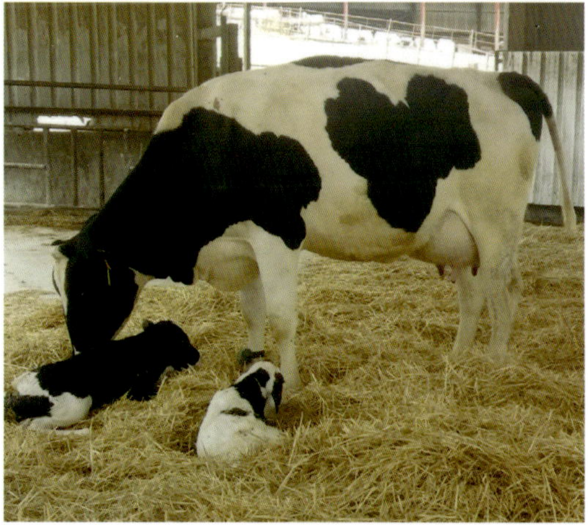

Figure 6. Straw is an excellent substrate for bacteria.

Compost bedded pack barns

This is an excellent solution to the problems seen with straw yard housing. The resting area tends to be made much bigger by incorporating the yard area. The bedding material is usually straw or sawdust which is aerated daily by a machine (rotavator, cultivator, harrow, etc.) and it is not necessary to add any more bedding (unlike a straw yard system), except when humidity is high.

The purpose of a compost bedded pack system is to reduce humidity, and keep the temperature, to approximately 20–22 °C, compared to the 30–32 °C for straw yard system.

This system can reduce new infections in freshly calved cows, as well as cases of clinical mastitis after calving.

Compost bedded pack barns prevent IMIs during the dry period.

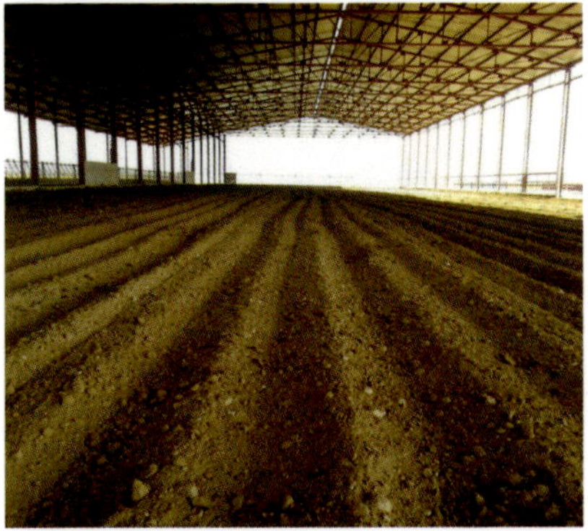

Figure 7. Compost bedded pack barns are aerated daily to reduce the moisture and temperature of the bedding, which reduces pathogens levels.

Precalving milking

This is when the cow is milked in the days prior to calving. It is not a very common practice, especially on large farms. This milking starts to prepare the udder, and improves teat hygiene and disinfection.

Objectives of precalving milking:

- Reduce inflammation in the udder before calving, reducing intramammary pressure.
- Reduce udder oedema.
- Flush out any microorganisms that there might be in the teat canal. The teat is more vulnerable, as the intramammary pressure precalving shortens and dilates the teat canal. The keratin plug also does not always form in some cows.
- Increase teat hygiene by washing and drying the teat before milking, milking and, finally, dipping the teat after milking.
- Rule out the presence of antibiotics. The first milk of a dry cow may contain antibiotics, so it is advisable to carry out a microbial inhibitor test.

It is advisable to carry out a microbial inhibitor test on the first precalving milk.

Precalving milking prevents mastitis and udder oedema. It is also important to keep frozen colostrum in stock on the farm, as cows that are milked before calving will not have enough. Precalving milking does not affect metabolic diseases, such as ketosis and hypocalcaemia, so it is not detrimental to cow health.

Epidemiological control during the dry period

Some tools are required to assess the state or level of mastitis in the herd at all times. Individual SCCs and good record keeping for clinical mastitis are essential to monitor the dry period, to maintain an epidemiological overview. These data should obviously form part of a herd programme to manage milk quality.

All the information recorded is processed, and udder health indices calculated. These are epidemiological rates or indices of mastitis, during the dry period in this case. Table 3 shows the results from a commercial farm, as an example.

Table 2. Udder health indices during the dry period.

Index	Parameter analysed	Objective
Rate of IMI at drying-off	Cows infected at drying-off	<20 %
Rate of new infections at calving	Healthy cows at drying-off that are infected at calving	<15 %
Rate of chronic infections during the dry period	Infected cows at drying-off that are infected at calving	<10 %
Rate of new infections in heifers	Infected heifers at calving	<10 %
Rate of cure at drying-off	Infected cows at drying-off that are healthy at calving	<70 %

Healthy: SCC <200,000 cells/ml

Infected: SCC >200,000 cells/ml

Table 3. Example of data collected on a dairy farm to control intramammary infections.

Date of milk recording	12/9/17	17/8/17	1/7/17	21/6/17	24/5/17	24/4/17	Average
Total dry cows	16	33	-	16	15	11	18.2
Healthy cows at drying-off	10	25	-	9	9	11	12.8
Infected cows at drying-off	6	8	-	7	6	-	5.4
New infections	1/10 10.00 %	3/25 12.00 %	-	3/9 33.33 %	1/9 11.11 %	2/11 10.18 %	10/64 15.63 %
Cows with chronic infections	2/6 33.33 %	4/8 50.00 %	-	3/7 42.86 %	-	-	9/27 33.33 %
Cows cured during the dry period	4/6 66.67 %	4/8 50.00 %	-	4/7 57.14 %	6/6 100.00 %	-	18/27 66.67 %
Total heifers	11	15	-	2	8	4	8
Infected heifers	1/11 9.09 %	1/15 6.67 %	-	0/2 0.00 %	2/8 25.00 %	0/4 0.00 %	4/40 10.00 %

References

Berry, E.A., Hillerton, J.E. The effect of an intramammary teat seal on new intramammary infections. *J. Dairy Sci.*, 2002; 85:2512–2520.

Bertulat, S., Fischer-Tenhagen, C., Suthar, V. Measurement of fecal glucocorticoid metabolites and evaluation of udder characteristics to estimate stress after sudden dry-off in dairy cows with different milk yields. *J. Dairy Sci.*, 2013; 96:3774–3787.

Bradley, A.J., Green, M.J. Dry Cow Therapy - An Update. *Swedish Veterinary Conference*, 2007.

Bradley, A.J., Green, M.J. A study of the incidence and significance of intramammary enterobacterial infections acquired during the dry period. *J. Dairy Sci.*, 2000; 83:1957–1965.

Cullor, J.S. The role of vaccines in the prevention and moderation of clinical mastitis. *Proc. 30th Annual Meeting National Mastitis Council*, 1991.

Dingwell, R. T., Leslie, K. E., Schukken, Y. H. Association of cow and quarter-level factors at drying-off with new intramammary infections-during the dry period. *Prev. Med. Med*, 2004; 63:75–89.

Dingwell, R. T., Timms, L.L., Sargeant, J.M. The association of teat canal closure and other risk factors for new dry intramammary infections. *Proc. 42st Annual Meeting National Mastitis Council*, 2003.

Dingwell R. T. *Strategies for the prevention and elimination of intramammary infections in non-lactating dairy cows*. DVSc Thesis. University of Guelph, Guelph, Ontario, 2002b.

Eberhart, R.J. Management of dry cows to reduce mastitis. *J. Dairy Sci.*, 1986; 69:1721–1732.

Godden, S., Rapnicki, P., Stewart. Effectiveness of an internal teat seal in the prevention of new intramammary infections during the dry and early-lactation periods in dairy cows when used with a dry cow intramammary antibiotic. *J. Dairy Sci.*, 2003; 86:3899–3911.

González, R.N., Cullor, J.S., Jasper, D.E. Prevention of clinical coliform mastitis in dairy cows by a mutant *Escherichia coli* vaccine. *Can. J. Vet. Res.*, 1989; 53:301–305.

Gott P.N., Rajala-Schultz, P.J., Schuenemann, G.M. Effect of gradual or abrupt cessation of milking at dry off on milk yield and somatic cell score in the subsequent lactation. *J. Dairy Sci.*, 2017; 100:2080–2089.

Green, L.J, Green, L.E, Medley, G.F. Influence of dry period bacterial intramammary infection on clinical mastitis in dairy cows. *J. Dairy Sci.*, 2002; 85:2589–2599.

Hemling, T., Henderson, M. IDF *Symposium on Immunology of Ruminants Mammary Gland*, 2000.

Hogan, J. S., Smith, K. L., Todhunter, D. A., Schoenberger P. S. Field Trial to Determine Efficacy of an *Escherichia coli* J5 Mastitis Vaccine. *J Dairy Sci.*, 1992; 75:78–84.

Huxley, J.N., Green, M.J., Green, L.E. Evaluation of the efficacy of an internal teat sealer during the dry period. *J. Dairy Sci.*, 2002; 85:551–561.

Lema, M, Tucker, W.B., Aslam, M. Influence of calcium chloride fed prepartum on severity of edema and lactational performance of dairy heifers. *J. Dairy Sci.*, 1992; 75:2388-2393.

Manteca, X., Mainau, E, Temple, D. Problemas de bienestar durante el periodo seco en vacas de leche. *Farm Animal Welfare Education Centre*, 2015.

Natzke, R.P., Everett, R.W., Bray, D.R. Effect of drying off practices on mastitis infection. *J. Dairy Sci.*, 1975; 58:1828–1835.

Natzke, R.P., Everett, R.W., Guthrie, R.S. Mastitis control program; effect on milk production. *J. Dairy Sci.*, 1972; 55:11256–11260.

Neave, F.K., Dodd, F.H., Henriques, E. Udder infections in the dry period. *J. Dairy Res.*, 1950; 17:37–49.

Oliver, S.P., Shull, E.P., Dowlen, H.H. Influence of different methods of milk cessation on intramammary infections during the peripartum period. *Proc. International Mastitis Symposium, National Mastitis Council*, 1990; pp. 92–97.

Oliver, J. Dodd, F.H., Neave, F.K. Udder infections in the dry period IV: the relationship between the new infection rate and the daily milk yield at dry-off when lactation was ended by either intermittent or abrupt cessation milking. *J. Dairy Sci.*, 1956; 23:196.

Smith, K.L., Todhunter, D.A., Schoenberger, P.S. Environmental pathogens and intramammary infections during the dry period. *J. Dairy Sci.*, 1985; 68:402–417.

Smith, K.L., Todhunter, D.A. The physiology of mammary glands during the dry period and the relationship to infection. *Proc. 21st Annual Meeting National Mastitis Council*, 1982.

Smith, K.L., Oliver, S.P. Lactoferrin: A component of non-specific defense of the involuting bovine mammary gland. *The ruminant immune system*. J. E. Butler. New York, Plenum Press, 1981; p. 535.

Smith, A., Dodd, F.H., Neave F.K. The effect of intramammary infection during the dry period on the milk production of the affected quarter at the start of the succeeding lactation. *J. Dairy Sci.,* 1968; 35:287.

Soback, S.,Ziv, G. Winkler, M. Systemic dry cow therapy- a preliminary report. *J. Dairy Sci.,* 1990; 73:661–666.

Sordillo, L.M., Shafer-Weaver, K., DeRosa, D. Immunobiology of the mammary gland. *J. Dairy Sci.*, 1997; 80:1851–1865.

Tao, S., J.W. Bubolz, B.C. do Amaral, I.M. et al. Effect of heat stress during the dry period on mammary gland development. *J. Dairy Sci.*, 2011; 94:5976–5986.

Timms, L.L. Field trial for evaluation of a persistent barrier teat dip for preventing mastitis during the dry period and as a potential substitute for dry cow antibiotics. In: *Proc. 40st Annual Meeting National Mastitis Council*, 2001.

Todhunter D.A., Smith, K.L., Hogan, J.S. Environmental streptococcal intramammary infections of the bovine mammary gland. *J. Dairy Sci.*, 1995; 78:2366–2374.

Williamson, J.H., Woolford, M.W., Day, A.M. The prophylactic effect of a dry-cow antibiotic against *Streptococcus uberis*. *N.Z. Vet. J.* 1995; 43:228–234.

Woolford, M.W., Williamson, J.H., Day, A.M. The prophylactic effect of a teat sealer on bovine mastitis during the dry period and the following lactation. *N.Z. Vet. J.* 1998; 46:12–19.

Zobel, G., Weary, D.M., Leslie, K.E. Cessation of lactation: Effects on animal welfare. *J. Dairy Sci.,* 2015; 98:8263–8277.